First published in Great Britain 2002 by Gaskell and St George's Hospital Medical School.

ISBN 1-901242-82-X

British Library Cataloguing-in-Publication Data

A catalogue record for this book is available from the British Library.

Distributed in North America by Balogh International Inc.

Printed and bound in Great Britain by Specialblue Limited, London.

Gaskell is a registered trademark of The Royal College of Psychiatrists.

The Royal College of Psychiatrists (no. 228636) and St George's Charitable Foundation (no. 241527) are registered charities.

Acknowledgements

We would like to thank our editorial advisers, Nigel Hollins, Brian Matthews, Richard West, members of the Crime Project at One-to-One (Tower Hamlets) and the Men's Group at the Joan Bicknell Centre for helping us think of ideas for this book and for telling us what was needed in the pictures.

We were very lucky to have representatives from the Home Office, the Metropolitan Police, Dorset Police, Victim Support and VOICE UK, as well as several carers and supporters, on the book's Advisory Group. We would like to thank them for their time, which they gave most generously: Geoff Bradshaw, Stuart Goodwin, David Griffiths, Louise Heatley, Abigail Hollins, Peter McDonald, Pamela Pearson, Stephen Tones, Kyriacos Spyrou and Catherine Alton Williams.

Finally, we are grateful to VOICE UK for having the idea for this project and for approaching the Department of Health, without whose generous financial support this book would not have been possible.

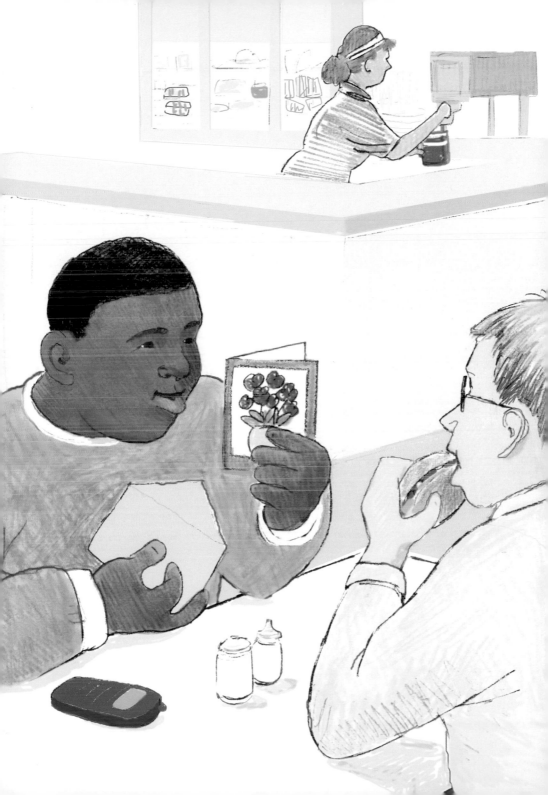

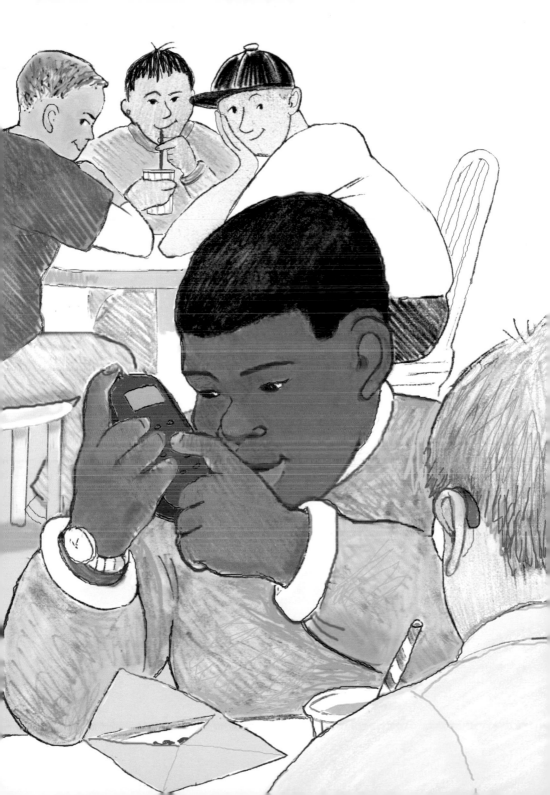

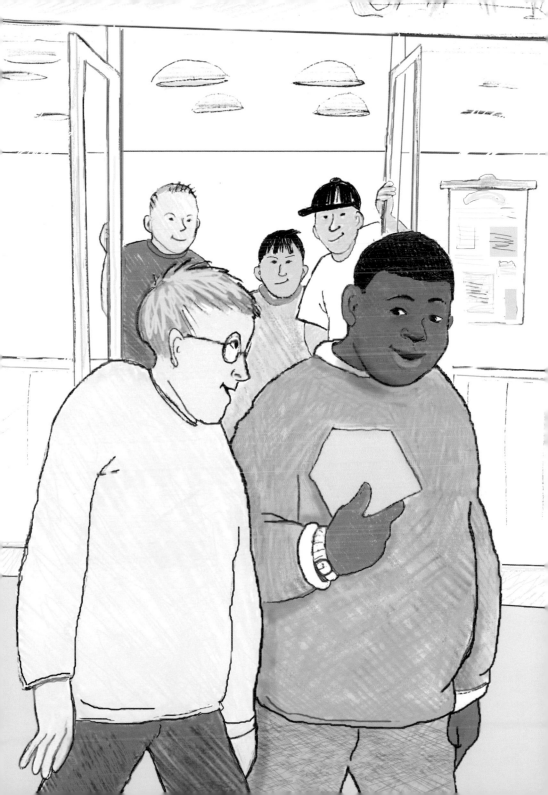

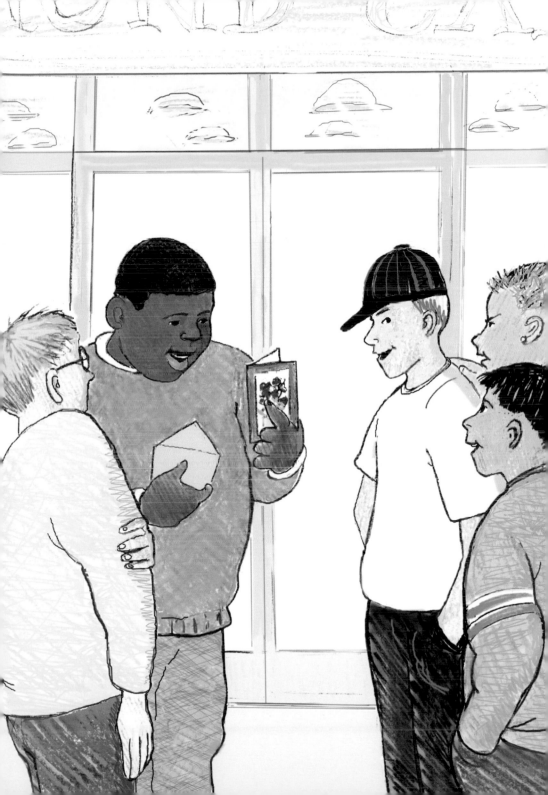

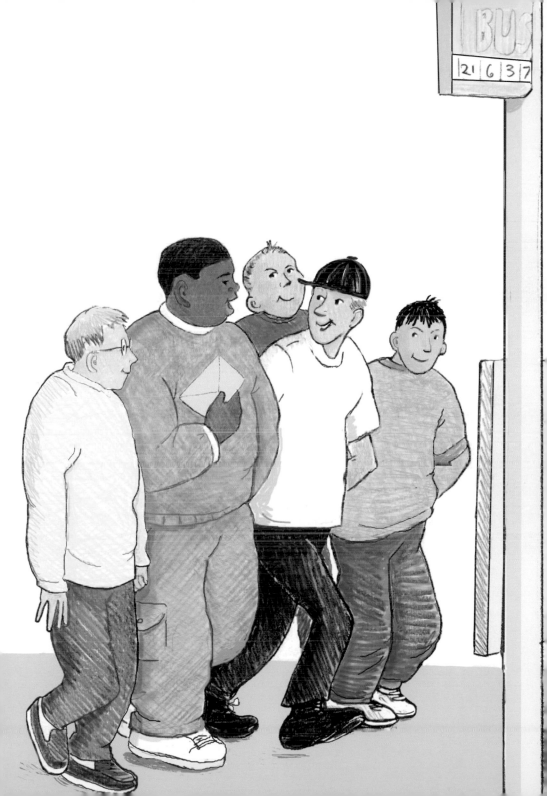

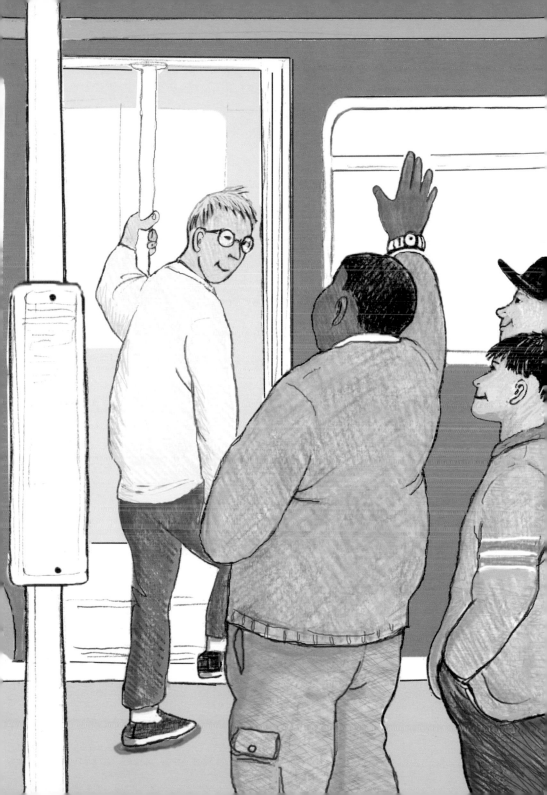

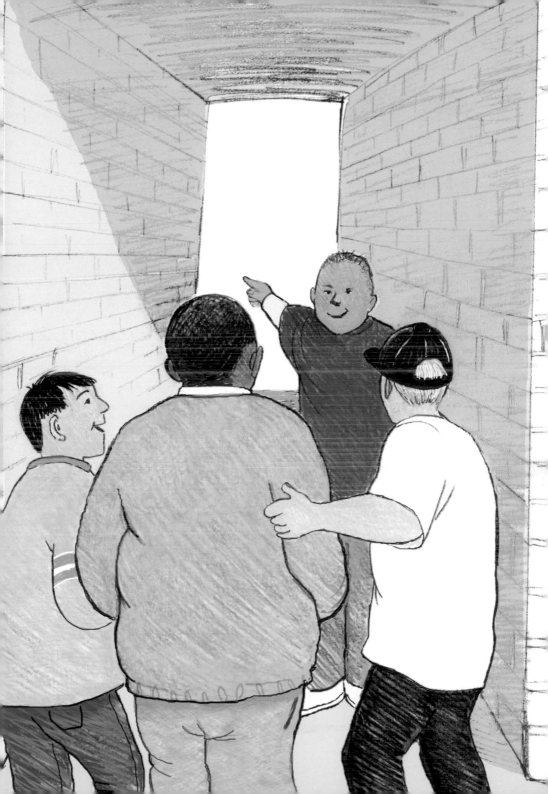

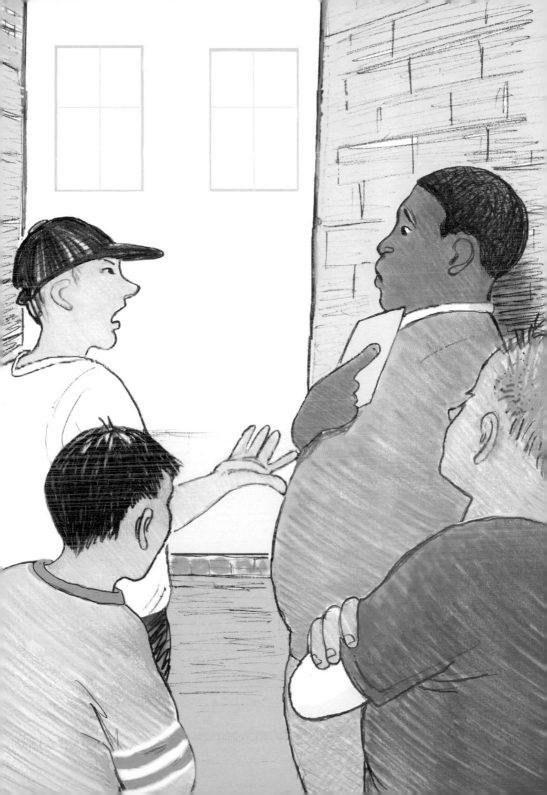

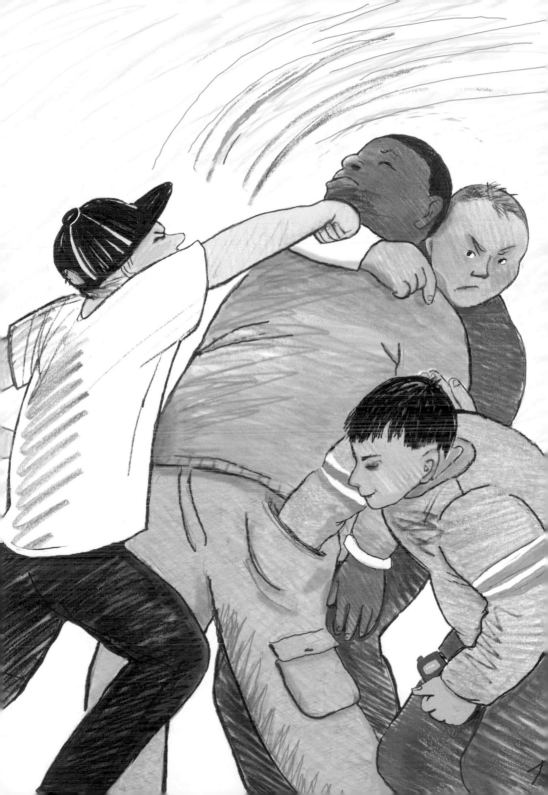

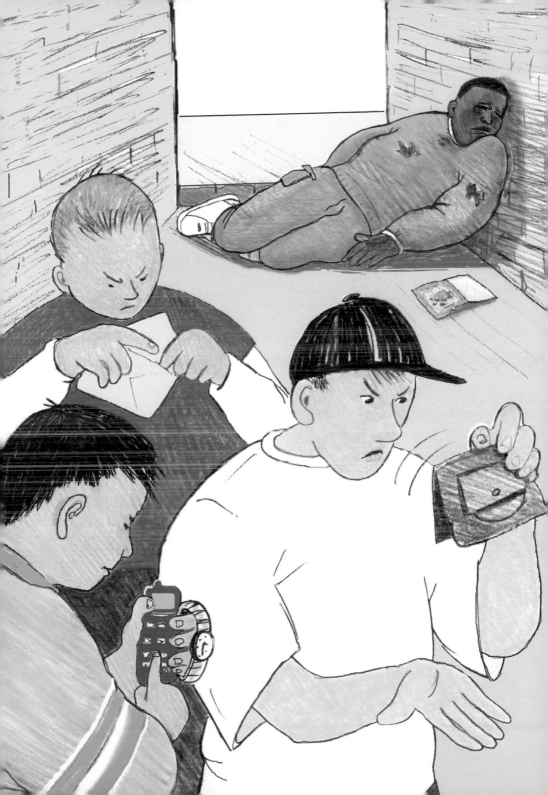

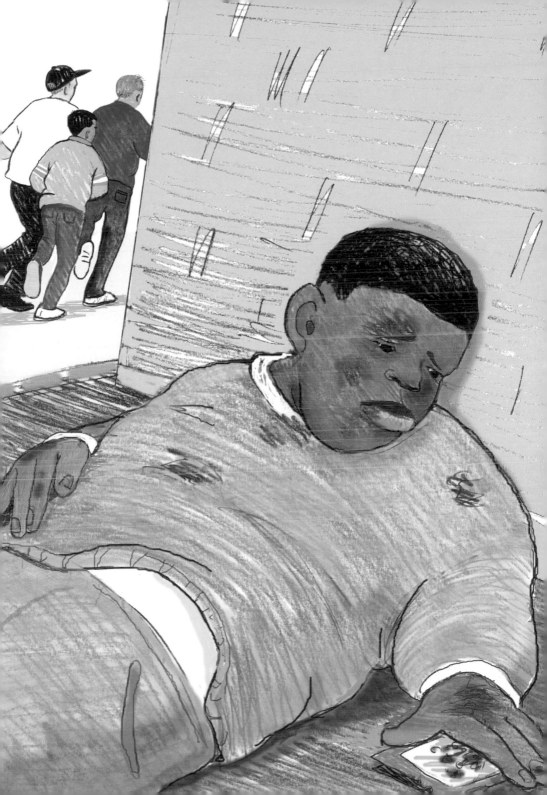

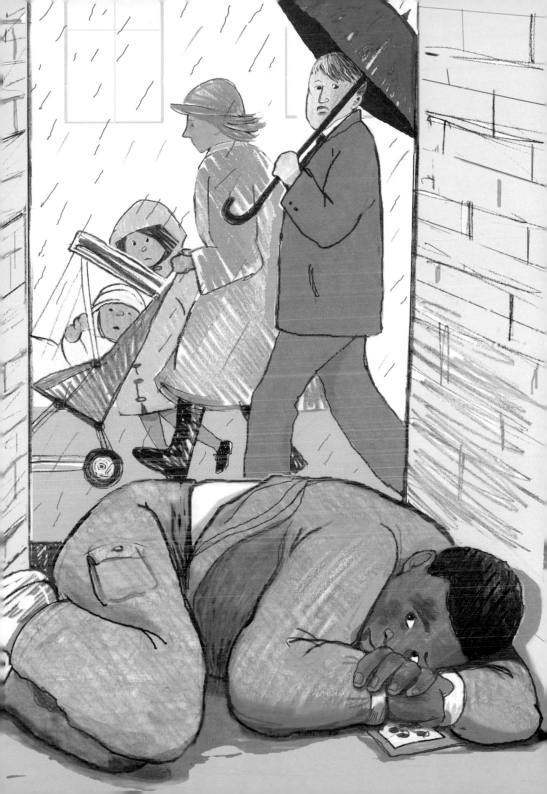

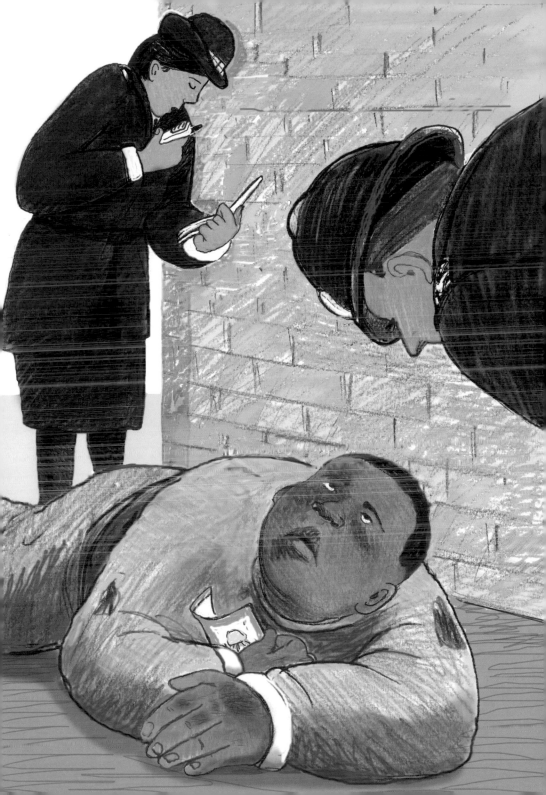

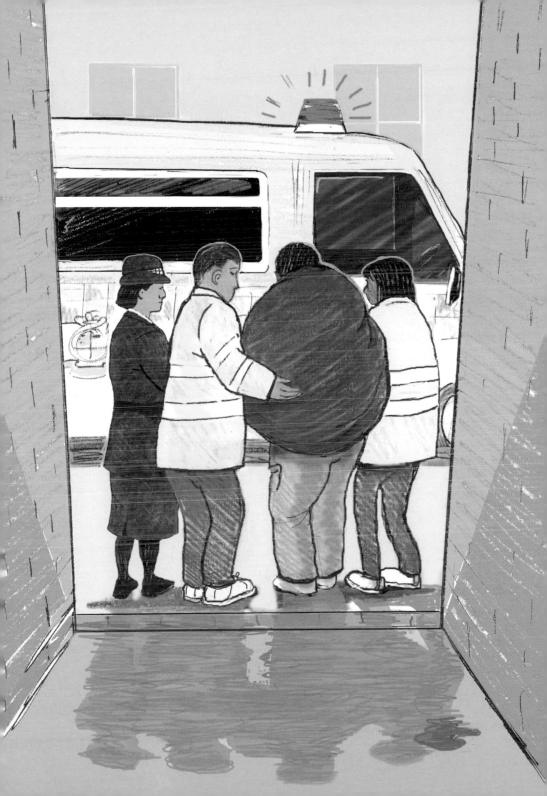

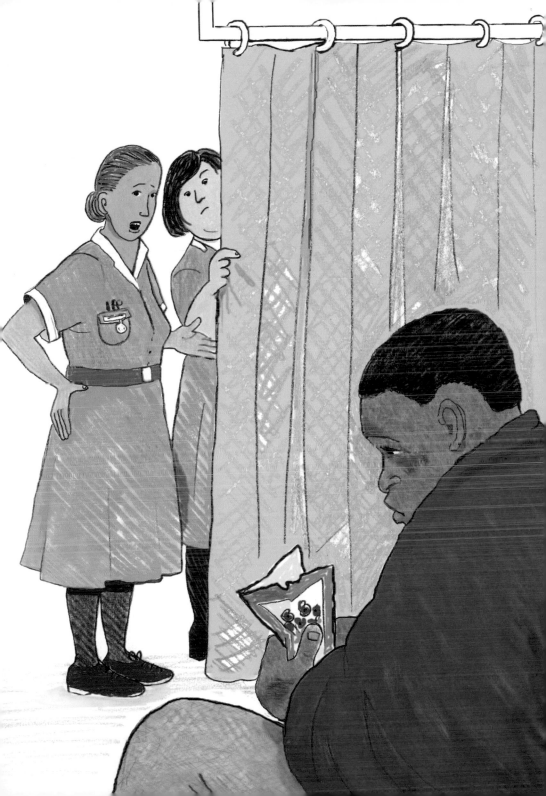

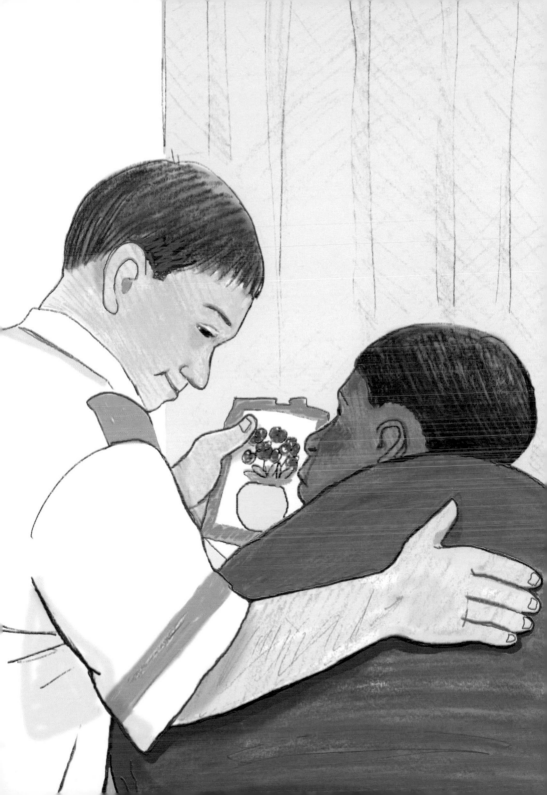

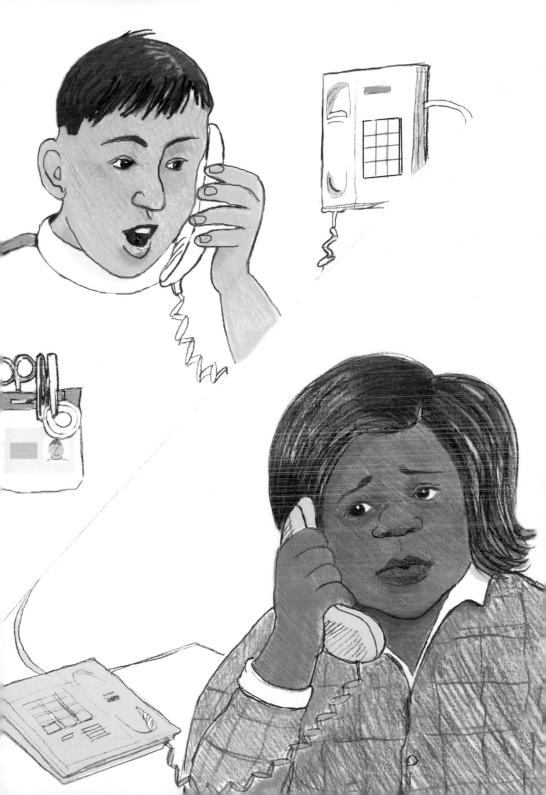

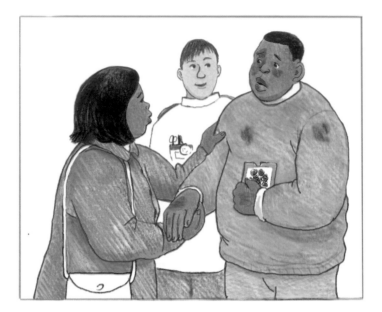

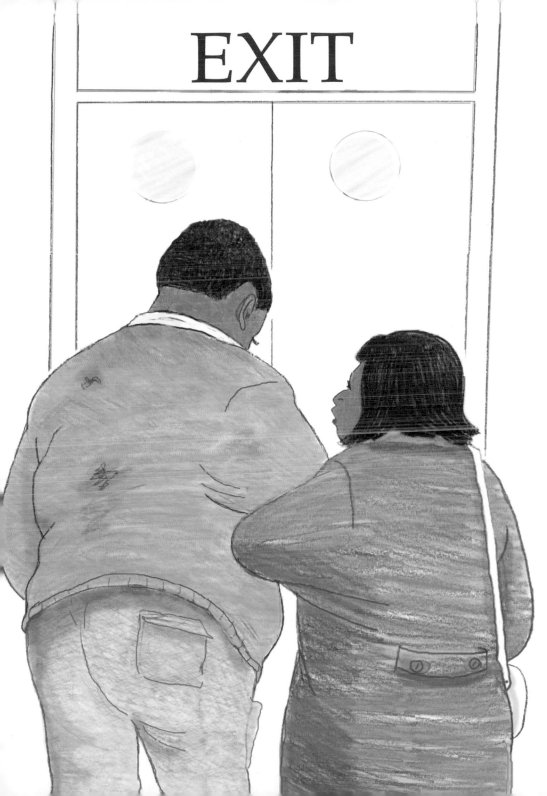

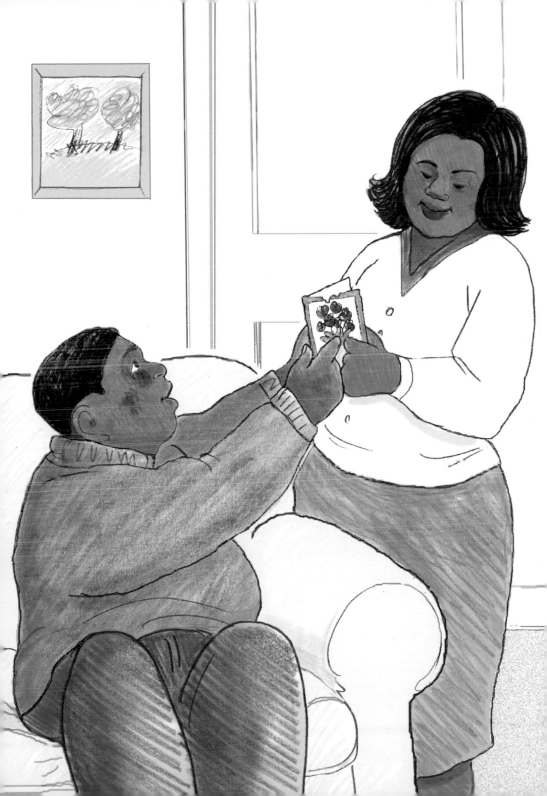

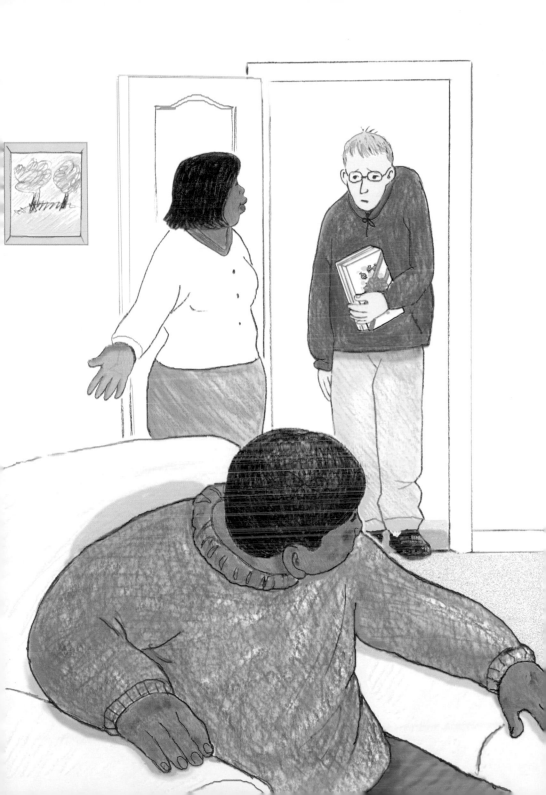

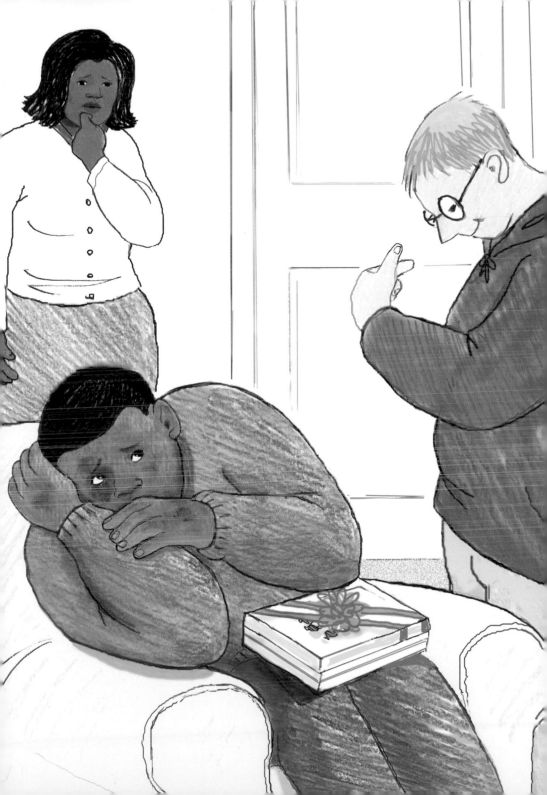

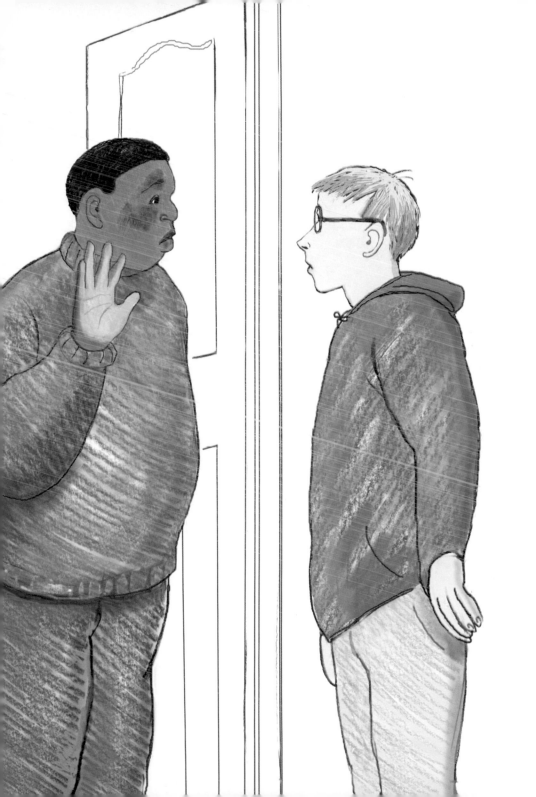

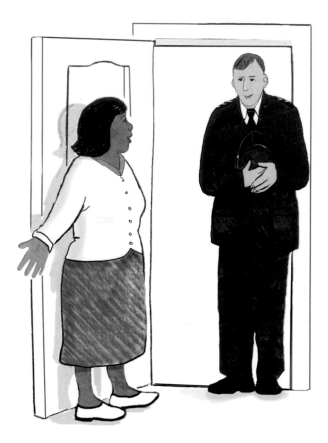

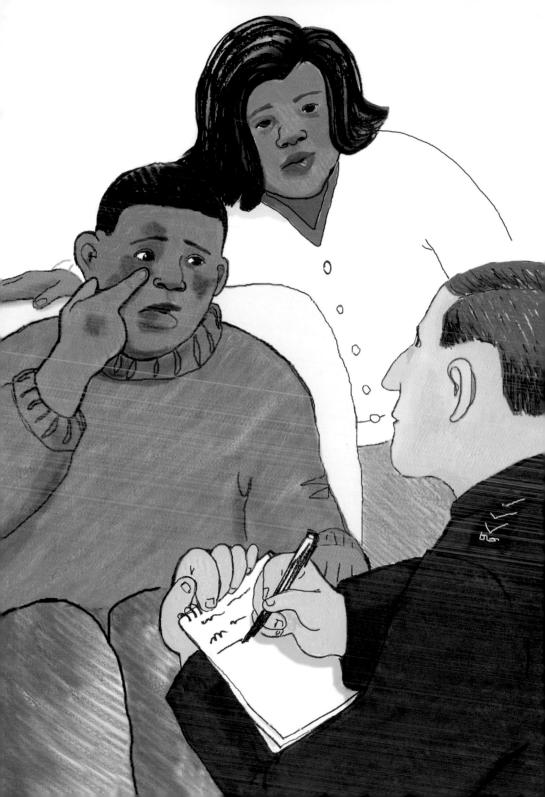

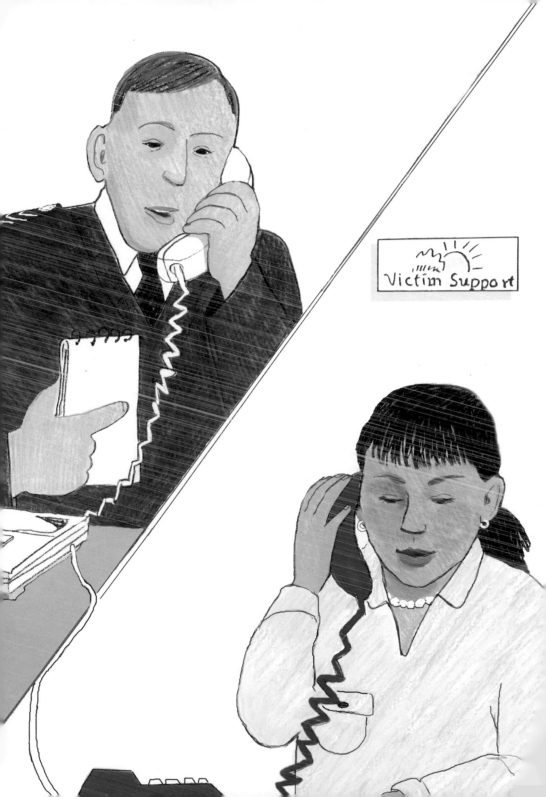

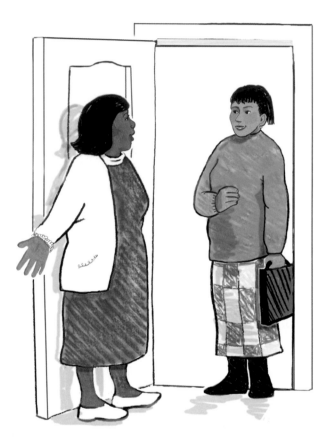

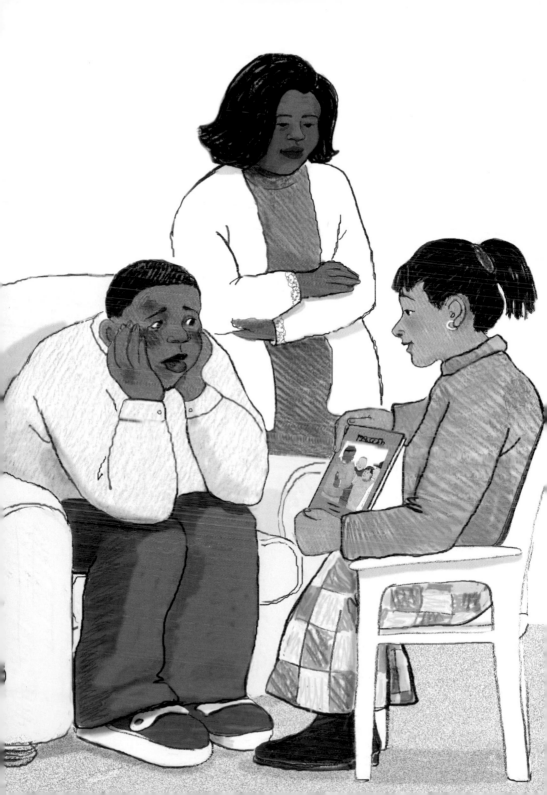

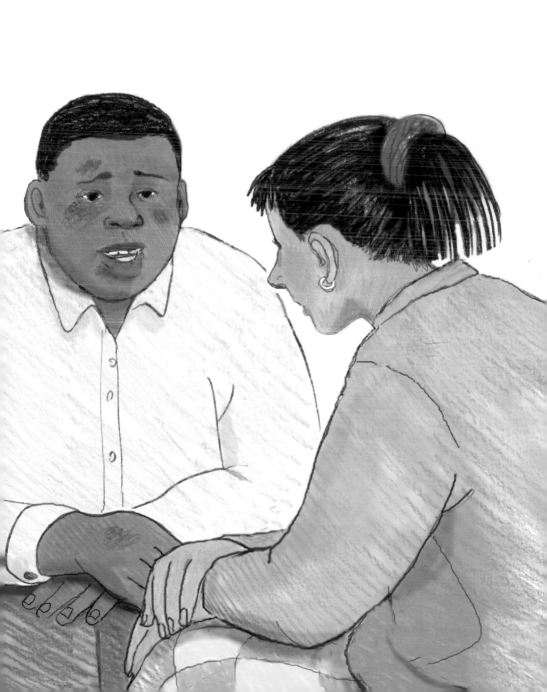

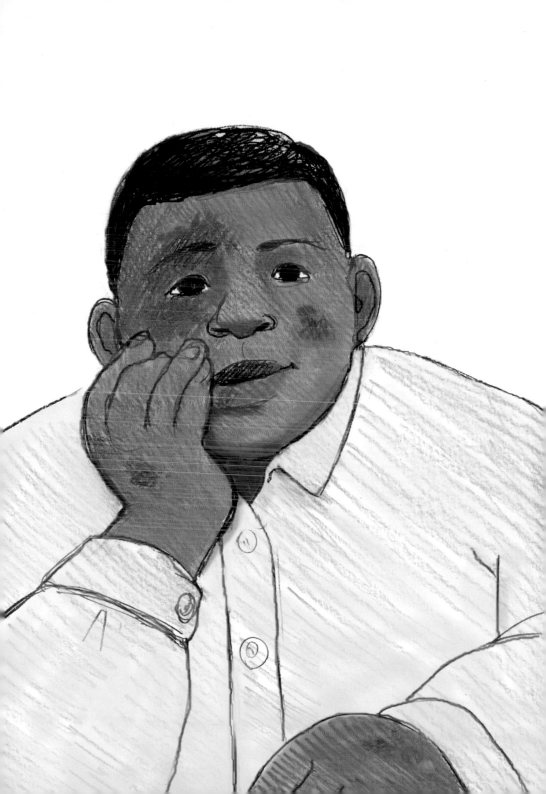

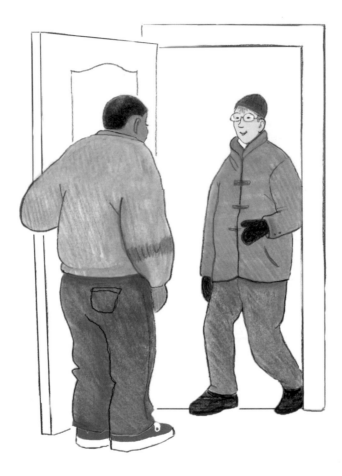

28

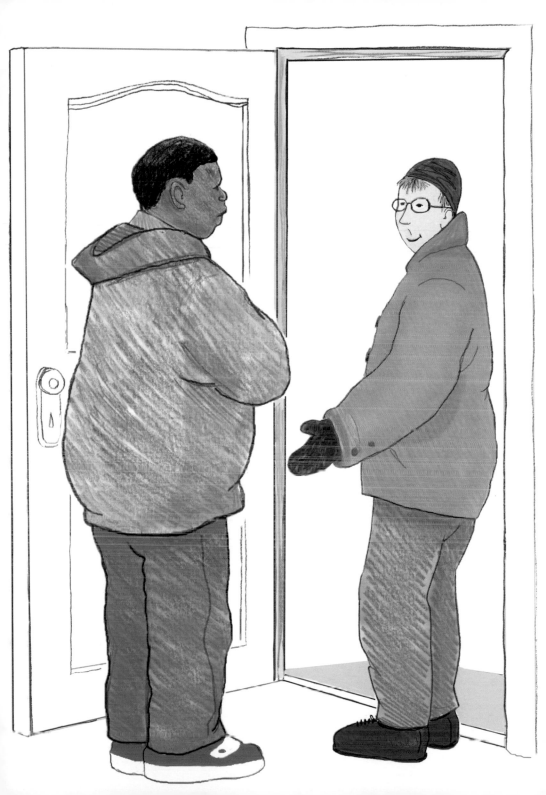

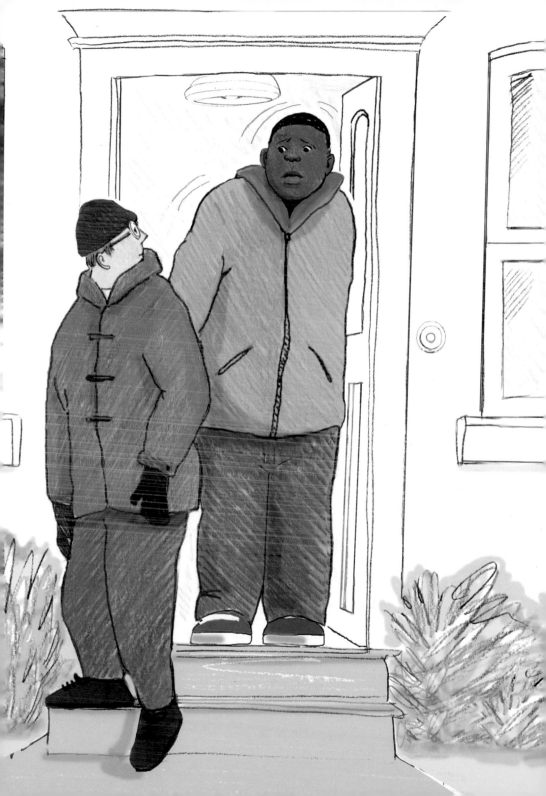

30

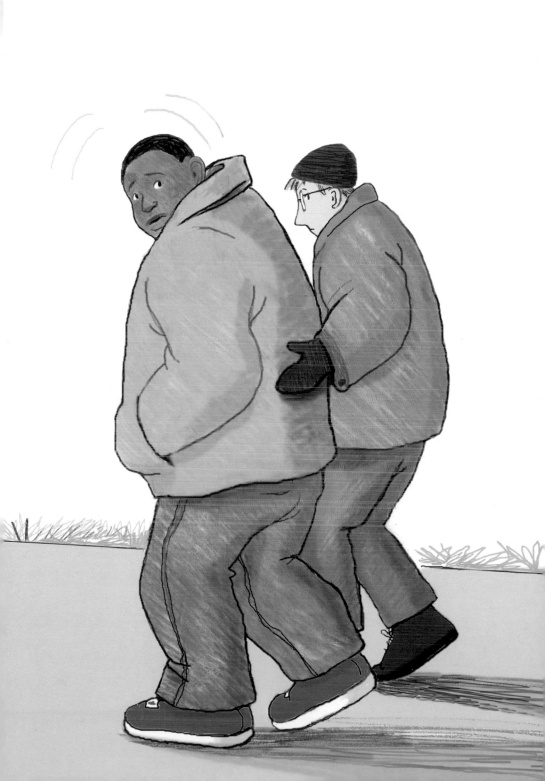

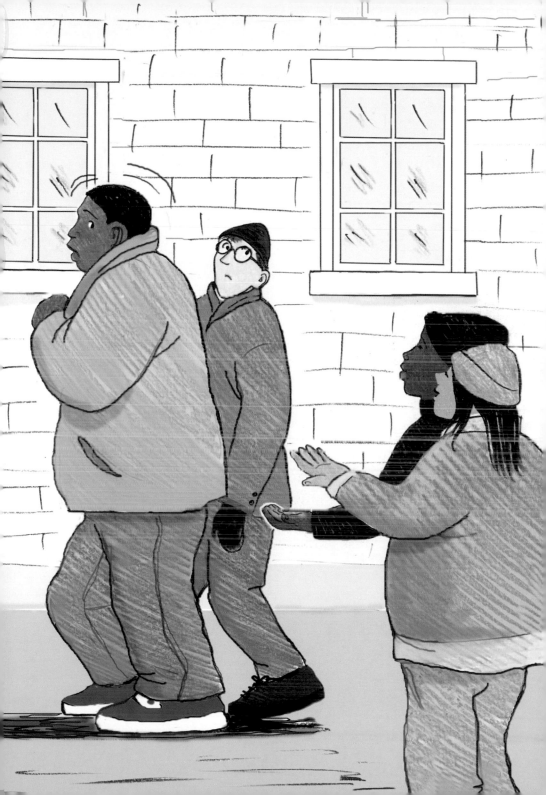

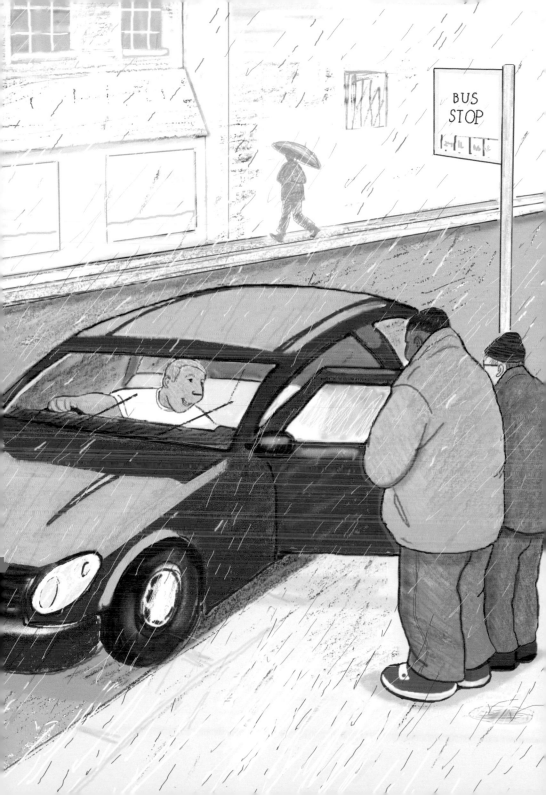

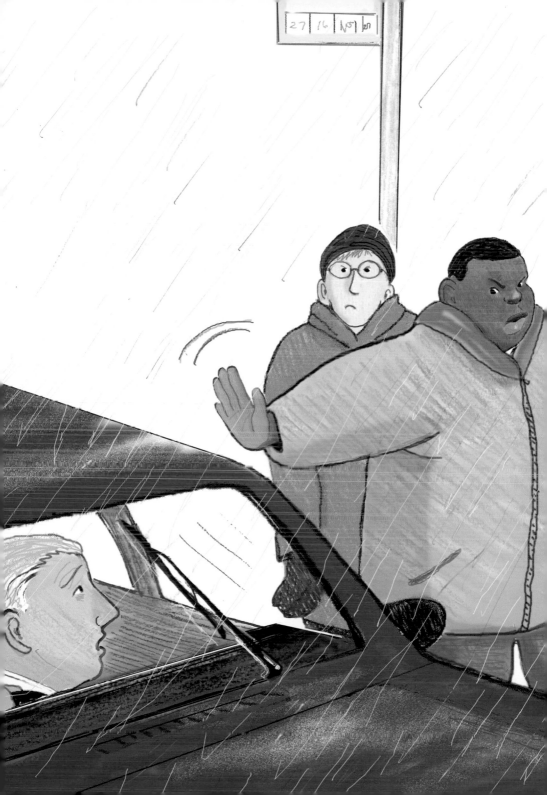

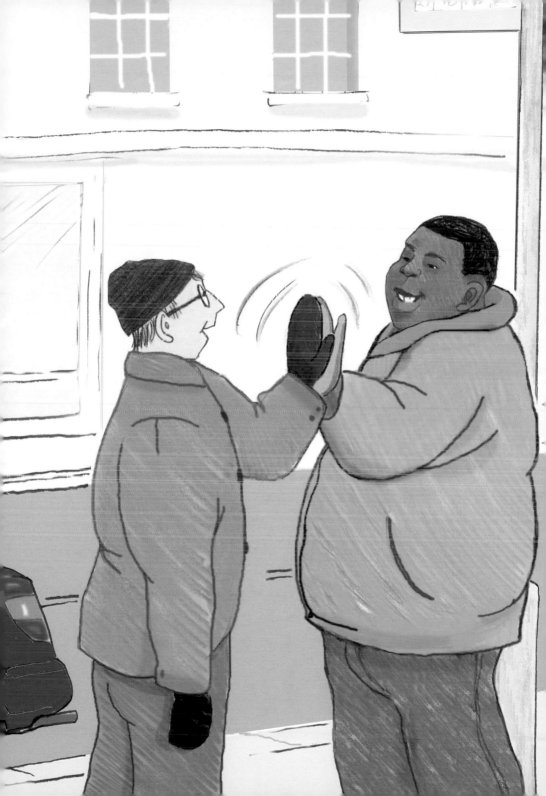

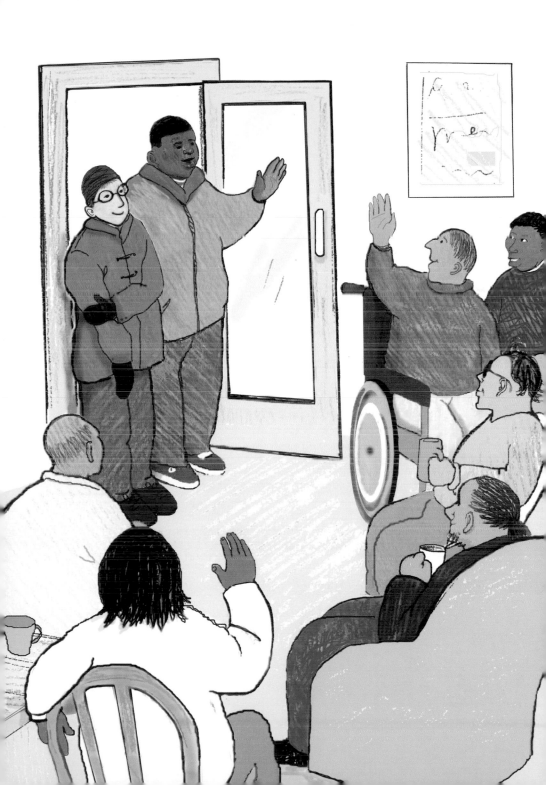

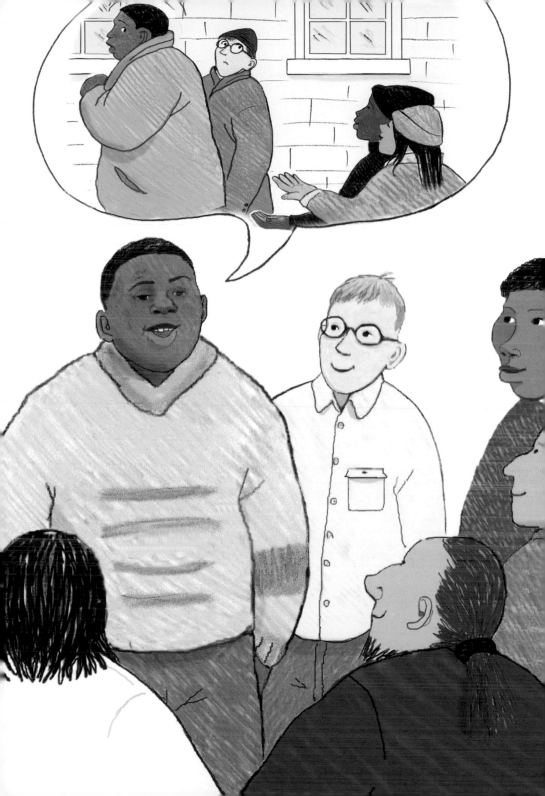

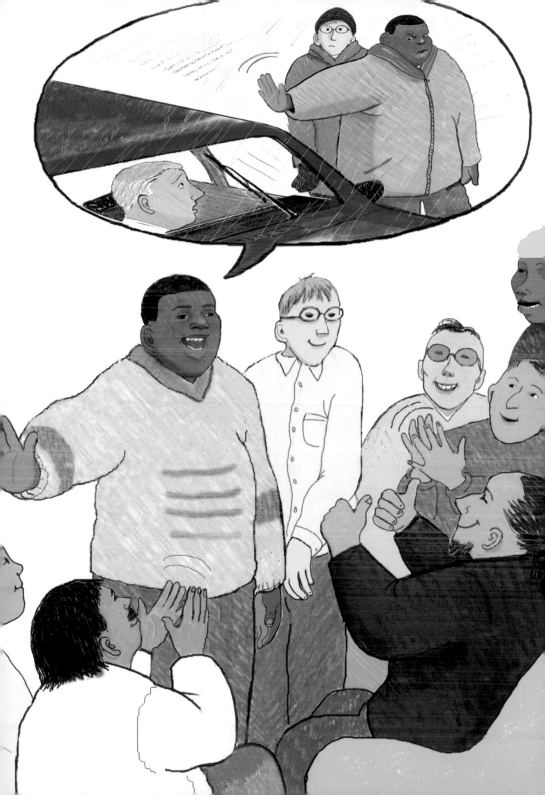

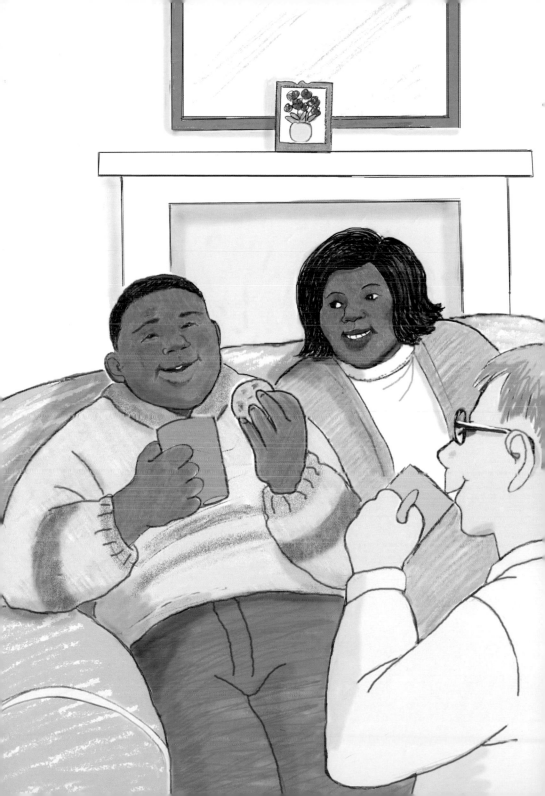

One man's story of being mugged

This story is about a man called Charlie. It begins in a café where he is meeting a friend. Charlie makes a call on his mobile phone. Some young men watch him, and follow him and his friend when they leave. The young men start to make friends with them, and walk with Charlie and his friend to the bus stop, where the friend catches a bus.

Charlie goes with the young men, who take him down an alley. They turn nasty and steal his mobile phone, his wallet and his watch. They hurt Charlie and run away, leaving him lying in the alley. Some people walk past, but do not know what to do when they see someone lying hurt. They get scared.

Two police officers find him there and call an ambulance to take him to hospital. The nurse calls his Mum, who collects him and takes him home. Charlie's friend visits him and invites him to go out. Charlie is too frightened to go out.

A policeman comes to take a statement. The policeman tells Victim Support what has happened to Charlie, and they send someone to talk to him about being a victim. He talks about his feelings and about being frightened.

After a while Charlie feels like going out again, but he is still a bit nervous. Some children approach Charlie and his friend, asking for money, and he is scared and hurries on. A man stops to offer them a lift while they are waiting for a bus. They don't know the man and they say "no". They meet some friends and tell them about how they are learning to keep safe. Gradually Charlie is getting his confidence back.

What happened next

The pictures in this book do not show Charlie's muggers being caught and charged. Also, they do not show Charlie going to court to give evidence. This book is based on a true story in which the man whom we have called Charlie did give evidence in court.

The people who hurt Charlie were convicted of grievous bodily harm with intent and attempted robbery. They were put in prison. This does not always happen. So how did the police catch them this time?

A policeman came to see Charlie to take his statement. Because Charlie had a learning disability, he had someone with him. He chose his Mum. Charlie took him to the place where he had been mugged. The policeman was impressed by how much he remembered. A lot of people, with or without learning disabilities, get so upset when they are mugged that they lose their memory about where the mugging happened. This means that some evidence can get lost. Sometimes people forget what the muggers looked like. Charlie remembered what the muggers looked like. The policeman showed him a copy of *Going to Court* – a picture book in this series about what it means to report a crime and be a witness.

Charlie had to wait a whole year before the case came to court. During this time he needed counselling to help him with his upset and anxious feelings. He kept *Going to Court* to look at when he wanted to. Shortly before the court case he visited the court to look round and practise saying the oath. Also, the policeman arranged for a short description of Charlie's special needs to be given to the judge.

Charlie was asked what it was like going to court.

Charlie: "I had to wait a very long time. The court kept on changing the date for the trial. It was a very important thing for me to do. I wanted to go to court. I wanted the judge and the jurors to know what happened. I wanted the men who hurt me to go to prison."

Question: "Did the barristers ask lots of questions?"

Charlie: "Yes. They listened to me."

Question: "Were you scared when you were being a witness?"

Charlie: "A bit. Just before. It was quite exciting being in court."

Question: "Were the men who hurt you in court?"

Charlie: "Yes – they were in the dock at the back of the court, but I didn't take any notice of them. I was looking at the jurors."

Question: "What did the judge say when you had finished giving evidence?"

Charlie: "He said I could stay if I wanted. I asked if I could go and he said yes. I wanted to leave it to the judge and the jurors. They all believed what I told them – that one man hurt me, and another took my mobile. Later my Mum said that the jurors decided they were guilty. The judge said 'Take them down!'"

Question: "Do you feel safer now that the men are in prison?"

Charlie: "Yes. I feel a bit safer, but I don't want to live in the same place now. I want a new home nearer to where my family live. I hope my new circle of friends will look out for me."

Unfortunately, the conviction rate following assaults on people with learning disabilities is very low. Hopefully, successful convictions like this, and changes in the law, should make it easier for vulnerable witnesses to give evidence.

Charlie had to go to hospital for treatment of his injuries. He has applied for Criminal Injuries Compensation (see later in this book).

Mugged

This book tells the story of a young man who is attacked in the street and has things stolen from him. But the story could equally apply to a woman. We are not sure how many people are attacked in this way every year because they do not always report it.

The book is not meant to scare anyone, but to help them deal with things better. This will mean that they don't need to be so worried.

Some people may need help to work with this book or they might like to look at it by themselves and then talk about it afterwards. They may like to practise some of the ways of coping, either with friends or in a group. As well as this book, there are videos, tapes and booklets about looking after yourself. Other sorts of training can add to confidence and self-esteem and make people feel less vulnerable. Some people might need help with going on public transport again.

This story doesn't explain what might happen if the muggers are arrested and taken to court. Our book *Going to Court* explains this very clearly. There have been some recent changes in the law to make it easier to give evidence. Details of these changes (called special measures) are described later in this book. These, when used together with *Mugged* and *Going to Court*, will help people to give best evidence.

What do you feel like after being mugged?

When you are mugged your world changes. You are no longer sure it is safe. It takes time to recover and you need friends and supporters to understand how hard it is.

If you are a man, like Charlie, you might think you should be very strong. To find out that someone else is stronger can make you feel embarrassed and angry. Some men pick fights to see if they have got any stronger. Then people get cross with them. They do not really want to pick a fight. They want to know that they are safe and have their self-respect back. Some men get very frightened and shy. Some hurt themselves and punch their heads. They want to be like the mugger and be the strong angry one, not the poor man on the floor who was kicked. So they kick or punch themselves. That too makes people cross with them. They do not really want to hurt themselves. They want to feel safe again and have their self-respect back.

It is easier to feel safe again when your attacker goes to prison. It can be a lot harder for people whose attackers never get caught. Then they can be frightened of going out in case they meet them again. People who are mugged sometimes feel too frightened to go out on their own. Friends can get cross with them and say they are cowards for not going out. But nobody has realised how frightening it is to see if the road is safe or not. If someone was mugged in a crowded noisy place they can find crowds and noise frightening because it reminds them.

Sometimes, people cannot enjoy watching television or going to watch a film. They cannot concentrate because they keep thinking of the horrible thing that happened. Sometimes, it keeps coming into their head like a bad film they cannot stop. Sometimes, pictures from it wake them up at night. This needs a lot of help and understanding so that people can enjoy life again.

Everyone needs to know that no one can be Superman or Superwoman. There will always be someone bigger and stronger who can hurt even the strongest people we know. When we realise that, we do not feel so ashamed. But at first some people blame themselves for not being able to stop it happening.

People think everyone will recover quickly. But it takes most people a long time. When a case is going to court it stirs everything up, and people who had got better can suddenly feel frightened again. Their friends and family need to understand this and respond calmly.

What was the mugging like? If a person or people quickly stole something from you, you might feel angry that something you valued has been stolen, but you might not feel very frightened. Being mugged means you are hurt as well as having something taken from you. Sometimes, muggers use words that hurt as much as their violence. Being called names or being laughed at can add to the feelings that you experience.

Once you have recognised the things that frighten you, and have been helped by friends and family, you will be on the road to recovery. If this does not work for you, perhaps because the feelings are so bad and won't go away, then you might need therapy. See our book *I Can Get Through It* if you want to know more about counselling and psychotherapy.

Some ideas for keeping safe

- If your pocket does not have a zip, somebody can steal your money or your mobile phone.

- If your bag is open, it's easy for somebody to take things.

- If you put your bag down and walk away, someone may steal it.

- If you go down an alley on your own, nobody will be able to see if you are in danger.

- If you accept a lift from a stranger, no one will know where you are. It is safer to say "no" – even if the stranger is friendly, and even if it is raining.

- If anyone attacks you, even someone you know, don't fight back. Do try to get away and report it.

- If someone snatches your bag, let it go and find someone to tell.

Role-play

Ideas for two people to act out

- Two people waiting at a bus stop, and one of them asks the time.

- Two people waiting at a bus stop. They do not know each other. One invites the other to go to his or her house.

- One person walking along the street. A stranger in a car stops to offer a lift.

- One person is looking in a shop window. A passer-by snatches their bag.

Working with a group

Two people act out a scene. Then the rest of the group talk about what happened. Two more people are invited to have a go, trying out a different response.

Getting in and out of role

You can give the characters imaginary names and occupations, and say where they are going or what they are doing.

At the end of the role-play, everyone should call the characters by their real names, e.g. "Well done, Bob. You played Charlie really well."

Extra support for vulnerable witnesses

In the past some vulnerable people could not go to court to say what happened to them. They were not considered 'competent' to give evidence.

In 1999 the Government passed the **Youth Justice and Criminal Evidence Act,** which deals with vulnerable (and intimidated) witnesses and is intended to help them to give 'best evidence'. This Act knows that vulnerable witnesses *are* able to give evidence and provides for a number of things which will help them to do so.

People who are considered to be vulnerable are those:

- under 17 years old

- who have a mental disorder or a mental impairment or learning disability (which could include autistic spectrum disorders) that the court considers significant enough to affect the quality of their evidence

- who have a physical disorder or disability (which could include deafness) that the court considers likely to affect the quality of their evidence.

Therefore, people with learning disabilities can be given extra help. This is called 'special measures'. The court will decide whether or not a witness can have special measures (see the next page) and if so, which. Ask the police for details.

Special measures (extra help)

Screens These can be provided so that the witness cannot see or be seen by the defendant.

Live links This is a television link by which the witness can give evidence without having to be in court.

Evidence in private The court has power to exclude the public and most members of the press.

Removal of wigs and gowns The judge can arrange that the barristers and the judge him/herself do not wear wigs and gowns.

Video-recorded evidence The court can accept as main evidence a video recording made by the vulnerable witness.

Video-recorded cross-examination The court can allow a witness to be cross-examined (asked questions by the barrister) on video.

Intermediary There is a new person, called an intermediary, who will be appointed by the court to help the witness give evidence in court. This might mean explaining the questions to the witness or telling the court if a witness does not understand.

Aids to communication Witnesses can have help to communicate so that people can understand them better, e.g. an interpreter.

To understand the meaning of the words witness, defendant and other words used in court, please look in our book *Going to Court.*

Where to find help and advice

VOICE UK is a support and information group for people with learning disabilities who have been abused and hurt, and for their families and carers. VOICE UK has a telephone service and tries to answer questions and help people with their problems. The group organises meetings in London as well as teleconferences (telephone calls that link people all over the country) on topics of interest to parents and carers. VOICE UK sends out a newsletter three times a year which tells how other families are coping, as well as giving information on what is happening about services for people with learning disabilities. Some parents who first went to VOICE UK for help are now helping other parents. Calling themselves Parent Contact Points, they will talk with other parents who have just found out about what has happened to their son or daughter and feel that their world has been shattered.

VOICE UK is based at the College Business Centre, Uttoxeter New Road, Derby DE22 3WZ. Tel: 01332 202555.

Victim Support is the national charity for people affected by crime. It is an independent organisation, offering a free and confidential service, whether or not a crime has been reported to the police.

Staff and volunteers in local branches give emotional support, information and practical help to victims, witnesses, their relatives and friends. This help can include arranging visits to see the courtroom before the trial, information on preventing future crimes and help in filling in forms for criminal injuries compensation.

Victim Support also runs the **Witness Service** based in every Crown Court centre in England and Wales (and an increasing number of magistrates' courts) to offer help before, during and after a trial.

The Victim Supportline offers emotional support and information between 9 am and 9 pm on weekdays, 9 am and 7 pm at weekends. Tel: 0845 30 30 900 (local rate).

Victim Support also promotes victims' and witnesses' rights in all aspects of criminal justice and social policy by lobbying the government for legislative change.

The Association of Child Abuse Lawyers (ACAL) offers practical support for lawyers and other professionals working for adults and children who have been abused. PO Box 466, Chorleywood, Rickmansworth, Herts WD3 5LG. Tel: 01923 286 888.

Easy to read information

Stop! No More Abuse. To help people with learning disabilities look after themselves. Joint booklet from VOICE UK and CHANGE. Price £2.00. Available from VOICE UK and from CHANGE, Unit D, Hatcham Park Mews Business Centre, Hatcham Park Mews, London SE14 5QA. Tel: 020 7639 4312.

Action Against Abuse. Recognising and preventing abuse of people with learning disabilities. For service users and supporters and families. Available from the Association for Residential Care, ARC House, Marsden Street, Chesterfield S40 1JY. Tel: 01246 555043. Price for 3 packs £35.00, ARC members £28.00. Service users' pack £10.00 (all prices include p&p).

Going to Court by Sheila Hollins, Valerie Sinason, Julia Boniface & Beth Webb. This is a related book about being a witness in court. It is in the Books Beyond Words series (for details of Books Beyond Words, see later in this book).

I Can Get Through It by Sheila Hollins, Christiana Horrocks, Valerie Sinason & Lisa Kopper. Shows how a woman is helped to get through the experience of being abused with the help of a counsellor/therapist. Also in the Books Beyond Words series.

Bob Tells All and *Jenny Speaks Out* by Sheila Hollins, Valerie Sinason & Beth Webb. These two books may enable a person with learning disabilities to open up about their experience of sexual abuse. Both are Books Beyond Words.

An 'A to Z of Harassment' is available in *Let's Keep Safe* and *Let's Report It* by Hannah Sharp. Price for the set is £5.50 (plus £1.50 p&p) for people with learning disabilities and their groups; £6.50 (plus £1.50 p&p) for others. Available from Values into Action, Oxford House, Derbyshire Street, London E2 6HG. Tel: 020 7729 5436.

Supporting Best Evidence by Philippa Bragman, Elaine Parry Crick and Christiana Horrocks. A guide for supporters of people with learning disabilities who are witnesses within the criminal justice system. Price £5.00 (plus £2.00 p&p). Available from VOICE UK and CHANGE (addresses appear earlier in this book).

Further written information

Parents Against Abuse. Book written with the help of parents whose son or daughter has been abused. Helps parents with strategies on how to prevent abuse and how to cope if it has occurred. Free to VOICE members, £3.50 to others. Available from VOICE UK.

Living in Fear: The Need to Combat Bullying of People with a Learning Disability by Mencap. Available free from Mencap National Centre, 123 Golden Lane, London EC1Y 0RT. Tel: 020 7454 0454.

A Guide to the Criminal Injuries Compensation Scheme (2001) is issued free by the Criminal Injuries Compensation Authority, Tay House, 300 Bath Street, Glasgow G2 4LN. Tel: 0141 331 5579.

Compensation

The Criminal Injuries Compensation Scheme was established to enable victims of a crime of violence that occurred in Great Britain to claim common law damages. You do not need legal advice or representation to apply for compensation. If, however, you would like help with an application under the Scheme, you can get advice from your local citizens' advice bureau, law centre or Victim Support office (see previous pages). *A Guide to the Criminal Injuries Compensation Scheme (2001)* is available free of charge from the Criminal Injuries Compensation Authority, Tay House, 300 Bath Street, Glasgow G2 4LN. Tel: 0141 331 5579.

Other titles in the Books Beyond Words series

Three books cover access to criminal justice as a victim (witness) or as a defendant: *Going to Court, You're Under Arrest* and *You're on Trial.*

The difficult subject of sexual abuse is covered in *Bob Tells All, Jenny Speaks Out* and *I Can Get Through It.* Counselling and psychotherapy after sexual abuse are explained in the third title.

Using health services is explained in *Going to the Doctor, Going to Out-Patients, Going into Hospital, Looking After My Breasts* (about breast screening) and *Keeping Healthy 'Down Below'* (about cervical screening).

Feeling Blue aims to help people to understand depression.

Speaking Up for Myself shows how people with learning disabilities from ethnic minority groups have the right to challenge discrimination.

Michelle Finds a Voice explains methods of augmentative communication.

Peter's New Home and *A New Home in the Community* help explain about moving home.

Forming new relationships is the subject of *Making Friends* and *Hug Me, Touch Me.* The ups and downs of a romantic relationship are traced in *Falling in Love.*

When Dad Died and *When Mum Died* help people to understand bereavement.

Two books about personal care are *George Gets Smart* and *Susan's Growing Up.* The latter tells the story of a young girl's first menstruation.

To order copies (at £10.00 each; £9.00 each for 10 or more books) or for a leaflet giving more information, please contact: Book Sales, Royal College of Psychiatrists, 17 Belgrave Square, London SW1X 8PG. Credit card orders can be taken by telephone (020 7235 2351, extension 146).